Racial Injury

understand Racial Injury,The Mental And Emotional Injury Of Racial.

By

Nancy P. Jones

Introduction

Racial injury, or race-based horrendous pressure, is the aggregate impacts of prejudice on a person's psychological and actual wellbeing. It has been seen in various BIPOC people group and individuals, all things considered, including small kids. Racial injury can be encounters vicariously or directly.Racial injury, a type of race-based pressure, alludes to Minorities and Native people's (POCI) responses to risky occasions and genuine or saw encounters of racial segregation. Such encounters might incorporate dangers of damage and injury, embarrassing and disgracing occasions, and seeing racial segregation toward other POCI. Albeit like posttraumatic stress jumble, racial injury is remarkable in that it includes continuous individual and aggregate wounds because of openness and reexposure to race-based pressure. The articles in this unique issue present new applied approaches, examination, and mending models to challenge racial injury. The creators urge clinicians to foster socially informed recuperating modalities and strategically refined exploration and desire the consideration of public strategy mediations in the space of racial injury.

Table of content

Chapter 1

What Is Racial Injury

At the point when individuals are exposed to racial Injury, segregation involves perceived hostilities or different types of abuse or viciousness as a result of their racial foundation, which can prompt trauma. Racial injury, which is otherwise called race-based horrible pressure, is the arrangement of outcomes that happen when an ethnic minority manages prejudice and separation. It typifies the changed mental, mental, and close-to-home damage that is brought about by seeing prejudice and segregation and by encountering it firsthand. A racial injury might be individual to one individual, or a whole local area might encounter it simultaneously. Racial injury, or race-based horrible pressure (RBTS), alludes to the psychological and profound injury brought about by experiences with a racial predisposition and ethnic separation, bigotry, and can't stand wrongdoings. Any person that has encountered a genuinely difficult, unexpected, wild bigoted experience is in danger of experiencing a race-based horrible pressure injury. In the U.S., Dark, Native Minorities (BIPOC) are generally defenseless because of living under an arrangement of racial oppression. Racial injury is a certain result of industrious openness to oppressive conditions that inwardly, mentally, and truly crush one's healthy identity while at the same time draining one's methodologies for adapting. It is a life-changing and incapacitating experience that influences innumerable quantities of ethnic minorities over numerous ages. Sadly, the inability to consider the interrelationship between racial abuse and injury restricts clinicians' capacity to work successfully with many ethnic minorities who live in the midst of sociocultural circumstances that are harmful to their minds and spirits. In any event, when treatment is injury informed, it seldom commits satisfactory consideration regarding racial mistreatment and the unavoidable injury related to it.

Encounters Of Racial Injury

Separation can mentally affect people and their more extensive networks. In certain people, delayed episodes of racism can prompt side effects like those accomplished with post-horrible pressure issues (PTSD). This can seem to be wretchedness, outrage, repeating considerations of the occasion, actual responses (for example migraines, chest torments, sleep deprivation), hypervigilance, low confidence, and intellectual removal from the awful mishaps. Some of these side effects might be available in somebody with RBTS and side effects can appear to be unique across various social gatherings. It is essential to take note that not all like PTSD, RBTS isn't viewed as a psychological well-being problem. RBTS is a psychological and physical issue that can happen as a consequence of living inside a bigoted framework or encountering occasions of prejudice.

Where Does It Come From?

Racialized injury can come straightforwardly from others or can be capable inside a more extensive framework. It can come as the consequence of an immediate encounter where racism is instituted on you, vicariously -, for example, where you see recordings of others confronting racism- as well as sent intergenerationally. Trigger Admonition: The accompanying incorporates conversations of misuse, attack, and viciousnes

Instances Of Individual Racism

Following the Coronavirus flare-up in the U.S., there were almost 1,500 revealed occurrences of against Asian prejudice in only one month. Reports included episodes of physical and obnoxious ambushes as well as reports of against Asian separation in confidential organizations.

In 2018, 38 percent of Latinx individuals were obnoxiously gone after for communicating in Spanish, were told to "return to their nations," called a racial slur, as well treated unreasonably by others.

Throughout the span of one year, Twitter saw 4.2 million enemies of Semitic tweets in only the English language alone. These tweets included the enemy of Semitic generalizations, advancement of hostility to Semitic characters or media, images, slurs, or against Semitic paranoid ideas including Holocaust refusal

Chapter 2

Causes Of Racial Injury

Racial injury can be brought about by one intense experience of prejudice (e.g., sexual and racial badgering in the work environment) or by various, more unpretentious types of bigotry that aggregate over the long run (e.g., racial negligible hostilities). Racial injury can likewise be brought about by the two encounters of plain prejudice and secretive racism. Any kind of pressure or uneasiness around racial elements or treatment can set off racial injury. A few models include:

Openness to racial or ethnic generalizations: illustration of this is when scholastics or reading material affirm that a few racial gatherings are better or more regrettable at specific undertakings.

Fears about private well-being: An illustration of this situation is the point at which a Latinx individual feelings of trepidation about the name of an undocumented migrant or an ethnic minority fears maltreatment by police.
Seeing individuals from an individual's gathering getting misuse: This can be, in actuality, or through the media, for example, when a Latinx individual sees migrant youngsters in confines, or an

Individual of color sees a video of an unarmed
Individual of color being killed.

Maltreatment of friends and family:

This can remember assaults for accomplices, guardians, or youngsters.

Direct openness to bigoted maltreatment or segregation: This might be hearing bigoted generalizations at work or being the beneficiary of a racial slur.

Others not treating encounters of prejudice in a serious way: This might happen when individuals question on the off chance that somebody's experience was genuine.

The rundown of racial injury is limitless. Different models might incorporate verifiable injury, perceived hostilities, and encounters of living with imbalances, like admittance to schools and clinical medicines everyday perceived hostilities — Proclamations like "What are you?" to an individual with earthy colored skin, or "What nation are you from?" to a brought into the world in this individual nation, may slip through the cracks by a White individual offering the careless remark, yet they can be profoundly pernicious to the individual on the less than desirable end. The practically oblivious looks and body developments showing dread or watchfulness when an Individual of color strolls by are likewise perceived hostilities. In the event that these episodes were uncommon, they may be no biggie. In any case, they aren't uncommon, and they are knowledgeable about the setting of culture with profoundly implanted designs of prejudice that keep on leaning toward White over Dark and earthy-colored individuals.

Encounters of separation and predisposition

These encounters can begin early: being named a conduct issue in school for basically being an uncontrollable, little fellow due to an educator's oblivious racial predisposition, or experiencing childhood in a less beneficial neighborhood in view of the enduring impacts of institutional prejudice in lodging. Furthermore, they can go on through life: inconsistent admittance to advanced education; being denied open positions or disregarded for advancement as a result of cognizant or oblivious racial predisposition; experiences with police that are more successive and more full of chance for Dark and earthy colored individuals than for White individuals

The profound type of assimilation

Once in a while, the conduct Dark and brown individuals embrace to prevail in a predominately White working environment or to squeeze into a predominately White people group can include concealing their actual selves. They might wind up acting circumspectly, hiding their feelings, and controlling their responses to bigoted remarks. This can be a personal strain that adds to racial injury.

Backhanded encounters of racist

Like openness to media inclusion of demonstrations of viciousness against Dark, Latinx, Native, or other minority people. These occurrences are stunning in themselves — to individuals of any race. Be that as it may, they can be particularly agonizing to individuals who have had related encounters of bigotry and segregation and can distinguish unequivocally from the individual who has been harmed or killed. A demonstration of police ruthlessness against a Person of color or lady can set off strong, instinctive feelings in other Individuals of color. They find in the harmed or killed individual somebody who might have been their youngster, their sister or sibling, or their dad or mom. Their psyches flashback to other, comparative occurrences where common Individuals of color have passed on because of police or White residents, and to encounters in their own lives where they have felt undermined and apprehensive, caused to feel unwanted or excused as not exactly completely human. This empathic reaction to a circuitous encounter is called vicarious injury. We feel maybe we had been straightforwardly

Chapter 3

Effects and symptoms

The joint impact of these kinds of experienced prejudice and segregation can work to harmful degrees of stress. The body delivers a consistent stream of pressure chemicals to keep a hypervigilant state in response to past and expected dangers. Our psyches stay fully on guard as though we are in steady peril. Furthermore, it could be said, we are. Racism is genuine and it's overall us.

Those sensations of stress and dread are exacerbated by a general public that will not acknowledge the real factors of racism. Time after time, our issues with perceived hostilities and demonstrations of segregation are met with protectiveness and forswearing, or even with rage. The issue is in us, we're told. We're excessively touchy. Or on the other hand, there's one more judicious justification behind what has happened that doesn't have anything to do with race. So besides the fact that we feel the aggravation of the experience, those sentiments are frequently discredited, which just exacerbates us — more separated, less certain, more troubled, or angrier.

Racial injury is comparable somehow or another to post-horrendous pressure problem (PTSD) in its impacts on the body and psyche. Yet, not at all like PTSD, the reasons for racial injury are continuous. There is no "post" to the injury. It doesn't end, basically not in our ongoing society with its well-established frameworks of racial predisposition and isolation. Thus, any mending or security from the injury should occur while the wounds proceed.

Not every person encounters racial injury because of these profound wounds obviously. Certain individuals even add strength to them. They have flexibility grounded in profound poise, solid social associations, and profound pride in their identity

Among the people who experience racial injury, impacts might incorporate

- Physical and social side effects
- Rest issues
- Expanded liquor or medication use
- Weariness, outrage, peevishness, or hatred
- Conduct issues at the everyday schedule
- Shaken trust in fundamental convictions
- A reduced feeling of safety, trust, confidence, and control
- An uplifted feeling of cautiousness and doubt
- Doubt about individuals outside one's family or informal community
- Carefulness of foundations and associations (government, social administrations, police, partnerships)
- Aversion to danger and hazard evasion
- Evasion of new circumstances and facing challenges
- More prominent aversion to encounters of lack of respect or disgracing

Mental and physiological side effects

- Ongoing pressure
- A debilitated invulnerable framework
- Expanded chance of melancholy and tension
- A change in mind action to limbic framework predominance (profound and rash reasoning

Chapter 4

coping methods

Racial injury can negatively affect your personal satisfaction, so finding proficient help is a savvy move (to a greater degree toward this in the following segment).

Meanwhile, there are ways you can uphold yourself at this moment.

practice taking care of oneself
As a matter of some importance, rehearsing and taking care of oneself is critical. Racial injury can influence both your psychological and actual well-being, so it's vital to focus on things like eating consistently and getting sufficient rest.

The same goes for side interests or exercises
that assist you with feeling invigorated, whether that is perusing a book, doing a workmanship project, or going for a climb.

It could likewise merit investigating a few new limits around consuming virtual entertainment and news, as both can be wellsprings of troubling data

Investigate activism opens doors
As far as some might be concerned, associating with others locally and taking part in various types of activism can be a recuperating experience.

A 2019 paper Trusted Source in the diary American Clinician noticed that following the injury of internment camps utilized in The Second Great War, a few Japanese Americans found it enabling to request affirmation of bad behavior by the U.S. government.

As well as giving a feeling of equity and conclusion, it likewise permitted them to interface with their local area and track down having a place by celebrating tribal Japanese practices.

Going to nearby fights or local
gatherings can be an effective method for beginning to reach out. Simply be aware of your energy. This kind of work can be debilitating, so it's vital to in any case cut out time for taking care of oneself.

Interface with others
On the off chance that others have minimized your encounters of bigotry and the subsequent injury, associating with individuals locally who've gone through comparative things can be a wellspring of mending.

Individuals you meet can offer approval of your
experience as well as survival methods that have
worked for them

Taking care of oneself: Recuperation Plan Steps:

Racial Health Tool compartment.
Depict what you resemble when you are overseeing and answering prejudice and racial injury in a solid way.

Day-to-day Support of Centeredness.
List associations or devices that assist you with keeping up with your centeredness despite racism. Such things incorporate, yet are not restricted to: Assets on racial personality and racial injury.

Associate with companions who are similar or better ready to take part in discussions about racial mindfulness.

Participate in a petition, otherworldly practices, or utilization of mantras.
Participate in activism. Practice self-administration (for example smart dieting, exercise, and most loved exercises that assist you with feeling focused).

Triggers and Reaction Plan
List things or encounters that will quite often bring about racial injury side effects (for example outrage, seclusion, trouble). After everything or experience, recognize a particular centeredness reaction (for example calling a companion, writing in your diary, activism).

Early Admonition Signs and Reaction Plan
List early admonition signs that you are
encountering racial injury (for example body hurts,
weakness, nervousness, sadness, trouble resting)
and related approaches to adapting from your
Everyday Support of Centeredness adapting
abilities list

Intense Racial Injury Reaction Plan

List signs that you are encountering intense racial injury (for example hypervigilance; uplifted close-to-home encounters, like sorrow, uneasiness, and outrage, which undermine your capacity to participate in picked exercises of work, rest, or school). Recognize an activity plan for everything on your rundown.

Emergency Arranging

Inquire as to whether you were encountering an emergency because of racism (for example contemplations of mischief to other people/or self; powerlessness to really focus on self as well as others; intense racial injury side effects that last longer than a predetermined term). List a person(s) or extra assets to contact on the occasion you experience such an emergency.

Post Emergency Arranging

List approaches to reconnecting with yourself and your networks to recapture centeredness despite prejudice and racial injury

Chapter 5

Five(5) strategies to support your healing journey

In this season of unbalanced Coronavirus passing rates, police severity, and People of color being in excess of multiple times bound to bite the dust in labor than white ladies, what does our mental mending resemble? The following are five techniques to help your recuperating venture.

Find the issue beyond yourself
Racism isn't your issue. Ever. By any stretch of the imagination. It is a successfully working framework that we, the African American population, and our partners are endeavoring to destroy. It is never your shortcoming. Let that go (actually quite difficult), and keep it moving.

Associate and reconnect with your racial character
The research proposes fostering areas of strength for an ethnic character .

safeguards against the impacts of the racial injury. This will appear to be unique for various individuals. It very well might be music, writing, visual media, food - any action that interfaces you with deep satisfaction in your way of life. For my purposes, as a Dark English lady of Jamaican legacy, paying attention to the music that associates me with my Jamaican culture has been vital - and not simply latently sitting back with music on behind the scenes, but effectively paying attention to the verses, hearing the crude importance in the verse. "Liberate yourself from mental subjection, none yet ourselves can free our psyche," has hit a specific harmony with me as of now.

Honor your assets and capacities

Racism is intended to work in a manner that can steadily, yet persistently, work on your confidence and fearlessness. We should act contrary to this. Question those self-questions by asking yourself where that belittling might originate from, and investigate an elective story that could serve you better. Encircle yourself with tokens of your accomplishments, concentrate profoundly on additional refining the things that you are great at, and invest energy with individuals who celebrate you in the fullest articulation of your Dark self

Recover your time, and use it to rest
This is a long, hard battle for Individuals of color -
it's nothing unexpected we feel depleted. We are
depleted in ourselves, and furthermore
encountering aggregate fatigue as a local area. To
continue to draw in or withdraw in this battle - in
light of the fact that both require exertion - we
should support ourselves. We should rest.

Utilize the aggregate ability to drive progress
This fight isn't our own to battle all alone.
Regardless of whether you find yourself the main
Individual of color in your neighborhood local area,
we have been honored with a virtual local area that
is meeting up to sympathize with their aggravation
and change it into something delightful. Associate
with others that you believe you can connect with,
share the heap, and find strength in meeting up.

Chapter 6

Consequences of and Outcomes Associated with Racial Injury.

Individuals encountering racial injury might experience the ill effects of a wide assortment of mental as well as physiological side effects. Mental side effects incorporate nosy considerations, social withdrawal, hypervigilance, low self-esteem, stress, and misery. Physical and substantial side effects incorporate migraines and rest aggravations.

Side effects of a racial injury can emerge at whatever stage in life, yet the side effects of racial injury appear to vary across life expectancy. Preschool and grade younger students experience dread for the well-being of themselves and their parental figures. Center younger students can start to foster negative convictions about their racial gatherings and begin to feel irredeemable or potentially numb when they witness racially persuaded savagery in the media. Young people might encounter side effects like grown-ups, however, the size of the side effects is reasonably more noteworthy in teenagers; this more noteworthy force might be because of the significance of social consideration during this formative stage.

Chapter 7

Contentions Against Marking Racial Injury as a Psychological instability

While there are a few specialists who declare that it is critical to comprehend racial injury with regard to PTSD, different researchers caution against the results of categorizing encounters of racial injury into a PTSD structure. One of the worries voiced by individuals who stand firm on this footing is that many individuals who experience the ill effects of side effects in the wake of encountering racial injury wouldn't meet symptomatic models for PTSD. The racial injury just can possibly turn into a diagnosable type of PTSD when it is brought about by racial provocation in which the minority saw or encountered their life to be in harm's way accepted or were truly hurt, or observed a danger of or experienced sexual violence. A few instances of this sort of racial injury incorporate police severity against African Americans and disdain for wrongdoings perpetrated against Asian Americans after the Coronavirus pandemic episode. Certain individuals stress that not gathering demonstrative measures for PTSD would discredit individuals' encounters of racial injury — possibly further worsening sensations of imperceptibility among racially minimized groups.

One more worry among individuals who are reluctant to mark racial injury as some type of psychological instability is that conclusions utilizing the DSM-V may mistakenly convey that such a determination exists inside the individual — instead of resulting from fundamental shortcomings. It can likewise leave individuals who experience the ill effects of racial injury side effects inclined to encounter both outer and incorporated shame in regard to mental illness.

Chapter 8

Contentions for Conceptualizing Racial Injury as PTSD

Racial injury is excluded from the latest release of the Demonstrative and Factual Manual of Mental Problems (DSM) since it doesn't meet the ongoing measures. racial injury brings out side effects like that of post-horrible pressure problems (PTSD), consequently the push for its acknowledgment as a feasible psychological well-being concern. The impacts race-put together horrendous pressure have with respect to people rely upon their encounters, and the manners by which it can show itself can change essentially as well. People who are presented with race-based injury or stress might encounter dissociative side effects following the event. Dissociative side effects incorporate depersonalization, in which a singular feels detached from their body or brain, and derealization, in which an individual has a stunning or twisted feeling of experiences.

Conclusion

At the point when it concerns racism, all things considered, not many individuals would be in question spot on and wrong. Except for fanatics, nobody would wish to embrace racism; pretty much we all know a terrible nasty racist way of behaving when we see it. However, there isn't generally lucidity about the most ideal way to answer, and not really certain about whether we might dare to fittingly answer.

It might shock you to discover that not every person would acknowledge us talking about racism regarding moral brain research or anything that approaches moral terms. For instance, some on the left of the political range would agree that racism is in a general sense political. Signs of racism are an outflow of a general public's progressive system: a method for a prevailing gathering or first class to keep up with its financial and social power. To allude to racism in some other term is evidently to overlook what's really important.

Some on the right, in the interim, keep up with that talking about racism- rather than racial bias or segregation - includes a vile disavowal of one's kindred citizenry. You might get down on nasty racist demonstrations or conduct, however, you ought to shun calling somebody a racist. The idea is that the last option includes judgments of a moral person, which probably places somebody shockingly awful of cultivated society. Obviously, I don't buy into both of these perspectives. While racism will have primary characteristics, it appears to be perplexing to dismiss the attitudinal elements of racial separation. For then, at that point, it turns out to be too simple only to fault "the framework", regardless. There can never be any liability credited to racism- you would never consider anybody responsible for nasty racism- in light of the fact that it is each a result of immaterial social and political powers. The people who demand perspectives assume no part overlooks the force of mentalities in forming social reality.

www.ingramcontent.com/pod-product-compliance
Lightning Source LLC
Chambersburg PA
CBHW061559250726

48657CB00021B/2393